Gut Health Easy Beginners Guide for Women

The Role of Gut Health in Immune Function

By

Brighton Archie

Table of Contents

CHAPTER 1

Introduction to Gut Health

The gut, also known as the gastrointestinal tract, plays a vital role in maintaining overall health and well-being. It is not just responsible for digestion and nutrient absorption; it is also intricately linked to various aspects of our health, including our immune system, mental health, and even hormone regulation. Understanding the gut microbiome is a crucial aspect of comprehending the complexities of gut health.

1.1 Understanding the Gut Microbiome

The gut microbiome refers to the vast community of microorganisms that reside within our gastrointestinal tract. It is a diverse ecosystem comprising bacteria, viruses, fungi, and other microscopic organisms. The gut microbiome is incredibly complex, with trillions of microorganisms coexisting and interacting in a symbiotic relationship with our bodies.

While the term "bacteria" might typically be associated with infections and illnesses, the majority of the gut microbiome consists of beneficial bacteria that play a crucial role in maintaining our health. These beneficial bacteria are collectively known as probiotics. They contribute to the breakdown of certain food components that our body cannot digest independently, producing essential nutrients and compounds in the process.

The gut microbiome starts to develop from the moment we are born, influenced by various factors like the method of delivery (vaginal birth or cesarean section), the environment we are exposed to, and our diet. During the early stages of life, the gut microbiome continues to evolve, becoming more diverse and stable as we grow.

The composition of the gut microbiome can vary significantly from person to person due to factors such as genetics, diet, lifestyle, and overall health. Certain bacteria may dominate in one individual, while different species may thrive in someone else. Nonetheless, a healthy gut microbiome is characterized by a balanced and diverse community of microorganisms.

Functions of the Gut Microbiome:

The gut microbiome performs several essential functions that contribute to our health and well-being:

1. Digestion and Nutrient Absorption: Certain gut bacteria help break down complex carbohydrates and fiber that our bodies cannot digest on their own. As a result, these bacteria produce short-chain fatty acids (SCFAs) and other beneficial compounds that nourish the cells lining the colon and provide energy to our body.

2. Immune System Support: A significant portion of our immune system is located in the gut. The

gut microbiome helps regulate and support the immune response, protecting us from harmful pathogens and infections.

3. Synthesis of Vitamins: Some gut bacteria are capable of synthesizing essential vitamins like B vitamins and vitamin K, which our bodies require for various biochemical processes.

4. Maintaining Gut Barrier Integrity: The gut microbiome contributes to the integrity of the gut barrier, preventing harmful substances and pathogens from entering the bloodstream and causing inflammation or infection.

5. Fermentation: Certain gut bacteria ferment undigested carbohydrates, producing gases like hydrogen, methane, and carbon dioxide.

While excessive gas can lead to discomfort, the fermentation process is crucial for gut health.

Impact of the Gut Microbiome on Health:

An imbalanced or disrupted gut microbiome, known as dysbiosis, has been associated with various health issues, including:

1. Digestive Disorders: Conditions like irritable bowel syndrome (IBS), inflammatory bowel disease (IBD), and constipation have been linked to an altered gut microbiome.

2. Immune Disorders: An imbalanced gut microbiome can lead to an overactive or weakened immune system, increasing the risk of allergies, autoimmune diseases, and infections.

3. Mental Health Issues: The gut-
    brain axis, a bidirectional
    communication system between
    the gut and the brain, demonstrates
    how the gut microbiome can
    influence mood, stress, anxiety,
    and even cognitive function.

4. Metabolic Disorders: Emerging
    research suggests that the gut
    microbiome may play a role in
    metabolic disorders like obesity,
    diabetes, and insulin resistance.

5. Skin Conditions: Skin health can
    also be impacted by the gut
    microbiome, with some studies
    indicating a connection between
    gut dysbiosis and conditions like
    eczema and acne.

Promoting a Healthy Gut
Microbiome:

Maintaining a healthy gut microbiome is essential for overall health and wellness. Several practices can support a balanced and thriving gut microbiome:

1. Consuming a Diverse Diet: Eating a wide range of plant-based foods, including fruits, vegetables, whole grains, and legumes, provides essential nutrients and nourishes the gut microbiome.

2. Probiotics and Prebiotics: Probiotic-rich foods like yogurt, kefir, sauerkraut, and kimchi introduce beneficial bacteria to the gut. Prebiotic foods, such as onions, garlic, bananas, and asparagus, act as a source of nourishment for these beneficial bacteria.

3. Minimizing Antibiotic Use: While antibiotics are necessary in certain situations, overuse can disrupt the gut microbiome. When prescribed antibiotics, it is essential to follow medical advice and consider probiotic supplementation to restore gut balance.

4. Managing Stress: Chronic stress can negatively impact the gut microbiome. Engaging in stress-reducing activities like meditation, yoga, or spending time in nature can promote gut health.

Understanding the gut microbiome is fundamental to appreciating the significance of gut health. The complex community of microorganisms within our gastrointestinal tract influences various aspects of our overall health, from digestion and nutrient absorption to immune function and mental well-being. By adopting a gut-friendly lifestyle, including a diverse and nutritious diet, probiotic consumption, and stress management, women can take significant steps toward promoting a healthy and balanced gut microbiome, leading to improved overall health and quality of life.

1.2 Why Gut Health Matters for Women

Gut health matters for everyone, but it holds particular significance for women due to several gender-specific factors that can impact their digestive systems and overall well-being. The gut plays a crucial role in women's health, affecting everything from hormonal balance and reproductive health to mental well-being and

immune function. Let's explore some
key reasons why gut health matters
for women:

1. Hormonal Balance: The gut
   microbiome has a direct influence
   on hormonal regulation. Hormones
   play a vital role in women's health,
   governing menstrual cycles,
   fertility, and menopause. An
   imbalanced gut can lead to
   disruptions in hormone production
   and metabolism, potentially
   causing irregular menstrual cycles,
   hormonal imbalances, and other
   related issues.

2. Reproductive Health: The gut
   microbiome can impact fertility
   and pregnancy outcomes. A
   healthy gut supports proper
   nutrient absorption, which is
   crucial for reproductive health.
   Additionally, an imbalanced gut

can lead to inflammation, which may affect the reproductive organs and overall fertility.

3. Menstrual Health: Some gut bacteria produce enzymes that metabolize estrogen, influencing estrogen levels in the body. Fluctuations in estrogen levels can affect the severity of premenstrual symptoms and menstrual irregularities.

4. Menopause Support: During menopause, women experience significant hormonal changes. A healthy gut can help support hormone balance during this transitional phase, potentially reducing the intensity of menopausal symptoms.

5. Digestive Comfort: Women are more susceptible to certain

digestive disorders, such as irritable bowel syndrome (IBS) and constipation. Maintaining a healthy gut microbiome can alleviate these uncomfortable digestive issues and promote regular bowel movements.

6. Immune Function: Women often have different immune responses compared to men. A balanced gut microbiome contributes to a robust immune system, reducing the risk of infections and autoimmune conditions that disproportionately affect women.

7. Mental Health and Stress Management: Women are more likely to experience stress and anxiety, which can impact gut health through the gut-brain axis. A healthy gut can contribute to

better stress management and improved mental well-being.

8. Bone Health: Emerging research suggests that the gut microbiome may influence bone health by modulating the absorption of essential minerals like calcium and magnesium. Strong bones are particularly crucial for women, as they are more susceptible to osteoporosis.

9. Skin Health: Women often prioritize skin health, and the gut microbiome plays a role in maintaining a healthy complexion. A balanced gut can reduce inflammation and skin issues such as acne and eczema.

10. Weight Management: Maintaining a healthy gut can support weight management efforts. An

imbalanced gut microbiome has been associated with weight gain and difficulties in losing weight, which can be of particular concern for women.

To promote gut health, women can focus on:

- Consuming a diverse and nutrient-rich diet, including probiotic and prebiotic foods.

- Managing stress through relaxation techniques and self-care practices.

- Avoiding the unnecessary use of antibiotics, which can disrupt the gut microbiome.

- Engaging in regular physical activity to support digestion and overall health.

- Seeking medical advice and support for digestive issues or imbalances in gut health.

By prioritizing gut health, women can improve their overall well-being, support their hormonal balance, and enhance their quality of life in various aspects. It is essential to recognize the unique connections between gut health and women's specific health needs to adopt a holistic approach to wellness.

CHAPTER 2

The Basics of Digestion

2.1 How the Digestive System Works

The digestive system is a complex and intricate network of organs and processes responsible for breaking down food into nutrients that the body can absorb and use for energy, growth, and repair. The process of digestion involves several stages, each facilitated by specific organs and enzymes. Here's an overview of how the digestive system works:

1. Ingestion: Digestion begins in the mouth, where food is taken in and

chewed to break it down into smaller pieces. Saliva, produced by salivary glands, helps moisten the food and contains enzymes that initiate the breakdown of carbohydrates.

2. Propulsion: After chewing, the food forms a soft mass called a bolus, which is then swallowed. The bolus travels down the esophagus through a coordinated muscular movement called peristalsis, which pushes the food toward the stomach.

3. Stomach: The stomach is a muscular organ that further breaks down the food through mechanical and chemical digestion. The stomach's lining secretes gastric juices, which contain hydrochloric acid and enzymes like pepsin, that

begin breaking down proteins into smaller peptides.

4. Small Intestine: The partially digested food, now called chyme, moves from the stomach to the small intestine. The small intestine is the primary site of nutrient absorption. The liver and pancreas release bile and pancreatic juices, respectively, into the small intestine to aid in the breakdown of fats, carbohydrates, and proteins. The lining of the small intestine contains villi and microvilli, which increase the surface area for nutrient absorption into the bloodstream.

5. Absorption: Nutrients, such as amino acids, fatty acids, monosaccharides, vitamins, and minerals, are absorbed through the walls of the small intestine and

transported to various parts of the body to support cellular functions and energy production.

6. Large Intestine (Colon): The remaining undigested and unabsorbed materials, along with waste products, enter the large intestine. Here, water and electrolytes are reabsorbed, and the waste material is formed into feces.

7. Elimination: The waste products, now in the form of feces, are stored in the rectum until they are eliminated from the body through the anus during bowel movements.

2.2 Key Organs Involved in Digestion

Several organs play essential roles in the process of digestion:

1. Mouth: The mouth is the starting point of digestion, where food is ingested, chewed, and mixed with saliva to initiate the breakdown of carbohydrates.

2. Esophagus: The esophagus is a muscular tube that connects the mouth to the stomach. It facilitates the movement of food through peristalsis.

3. Stomach: The stomach is a sac-like organ that stores and mixes food with gastric juices to begin protein digestion.

4. Liver: The liver is the largest internal organ and has multiple

functions in digestion. It produces
bile, which is stored in the
gallbladder and released into the
small intestine to aid in the
breakdown of fats.

5. Gallbladder: The gallbladder stores
    and concentrates bile produced by
    the liver. It releases bile into the
    small intestine when needed for fat
    digestion.

6. Pancreas: The pancreas is both an
    endocrine and exocrine gland. As
    part of the digestive system, it
    produces pancreatic juices
    containing enzymes that help
    further break down carbohydrates,
    proteins, and fats in the small
    intestine.

7. Small Intestine: The small
    intestine is a long, coiled tube

where the majority of digestion
and nutrient absorption occur.

8. Large Intestine (Colon): The large
    intestine is responsible for
    absorbing water and electrolytes
    from the remaining undigested
    food, forming feces, and
    facilitating their elimination.

Each organ in the digestive system
plays a specific role in the overall
process of digestion and ensures that
the body receives the necessary
nutrients from the food we eat to
maintain proper health and
functioning.

CHAPTER 3

Signs of a Healthy Gut

3.1 Identifying a Well-Functioning Gut

A well-functioning gut is essential for overall health and well-being. When the gut is in good condition, it efficiently absorbs nutrients, supports the immune system, and maintains a balanced gut microbiome. Here are some signs of a healthy gut:

1. Regular and Well-Formed Bowel Movements: A healthy gut typically leads to regular bowel movements that are well-formed and easy to pass. Bowel

movements should occur without discomfort or excessive straining.

2. Consistent Digestion: After eating, there should be a sense of ease in digestion. Meals should not lead to persistent bloating, gas, or indigestion.

3. No Unexplained Weight Fluctuations: A healthy gut helps maintain a stable weight. Unexplained weight loss or gain without changes in diet or activity levels may indicate an issue with gut health.

4. High Energy Levels: A well-functioning gut allows for efficient absorption of nutrients, contributing to higher energy levels and overall vitality.

5. Good Skin Health: The condition of the skin can be an indicator of

gut health. A healthy gut is often reflected in clear and glowing skin.

6. Balanced Mood: The gut-brain axis influences mood and emotional well-being. A healthy gut can contribute to a more stable and balanced mood.

7. Strong Immune System: A well-functioning gut supports a robust immune system, helping the body fight off infections and illnesses.

8. Healthy Breath: Bad breath can sometimes be linked to digestive issues, so having fresh breath can be a positive sign of gut health.

9. Minimal Food Sensitivities: A healthy gut can tolerate a variety of foods without causing significant sensitivities or allergies.

10. Optimal Absorption of Nutrients:
A healthy gut effectively absorbs
essential nutrients from the food
we eat, promoting overall health
and vitality.

Individual variations are common,
and what constitutes a healthy gut can
vary from person to person. If you
have concerns about your gut health,
it's always a good idea to consult a
healthcare professional.

3.2 Common Gut Health Issues for Women

Women may experience certain gut
health issues that are more prevalent
or have distinct features compared to
men. Some of these common gut
health issues for women include:

1. Irritable Bowel Syndrome (IBS): IBS is a functional digestive disorder that affects the large intestine and can lead to symptoms like abdominal pain, bloating, gas, and changes in bowel habits. Women are more likely to be diagnosed with IBS than men.

2. Constipation: Women are generally more prone to constipation, which is characterized by infrequent and difficult bowel movements.

3. Inflammatory Bowel Disease (IBD): Although IBD, including Crohn's disease and ulcerative colitis, affects both men and women, some studies suggest that women may experience more severe symptoms and specific challenges during pregnancy and menstruation.

4. Gut-Brain Axis Disorders: Women
   may be more susceptible to gut-
   brain axis disorders, such as
   irritable bowel syndrome with
   predominant diarrhea (IBS-D) and
   functional dyspepsia. These
   conditions involve complex
   interactions between the gut and
   the brain, often influenced by
   hormonal changes and stress.

5. Gut Health During Pregnancy:
   Pregnancy can lead to various
   changes in gut health due to
   hormonal fluctuations, altered gut
   motility, and potential shifts in gut
   microbiota. Some women may
   experience digestive discomfort or
   issues during pregnancy.

6. Gut Health and Menstrual Cycle:
   The menstrual cycle can influence
   gut health and vice versa.
   Fluctuations in hormones during

the menstrual cycle can impact gut function and may contribute to premenstrual symptoms.

7. Gut Health and Menopause: During menopause, women experience significant hormonal changes, which can affect gut health and lead to digestive issues such as bloating and changes in bowel habits.

8. Gut Dysbiosis: Women may be more susceptible to disruptions in gut microbiota due to factors like hormonal birth control, antibiotic use, and dietary changes.

As with any health concern, it is essential for women to be proactive about their gut health and seek medical advice if they experience persistent digestive symptoms or concerns. Maintaining a balanced diet, managing stress, staying hydrated, and leading a healthy lifestyle can all contribute to better gut health for women.

CHAPTER 4

Factors Affecting Gut Health

4.1 Diet and Nutrition

Diet and nutrition play a significant role in shaping the health of the gut. The foods we eat can either promote a healthy gut environment or disrupt the delicate balance of the gut microbiome. A well-balanced and nutrient-rich diet can support optimal gut health, while poor dietary choices can lead to gut imbalances and digestive issues. Here are some factors to consider for maintaining a gut-friendly diet:

4.1.1 Gut-Friendly Foods

1. Fiber-Rich Foods: Foods high in soluble and insoluble fiber, such as fruits, vegetables, whole grains, nuts, and seeds, are excellent for gut health. Fiber supports regular bowel movements, feeds beneficial gut bacteria, and helps maintain a healthy gut lining.

2. Fermented Foods: Fermented foods are rich in probiotics, which are beneficial live bacteria that promote gut health. Examples include yogurt, kefir, sauerkraut, kimchi, miso, and tempeh.

3. Prebiotic Foods: Prebiotics are non-digestible fibers that serve as food for probiotics, helping them thrive in the gut. Foods like onions, garlic, bananas, asparagus, and chicory root are excellent sources of prebiotics.

4. Lean Proteins: Consuming lean sources of protein, such as fish, poultry, tofu, and legumes, can support gut health while providing essential amino acids for the body.

5. Omega-3 Fatty Acids: Foods rich in omega-3 fatty acids, such as fatty fish (salmon, mackerel, sardines), flaxseeds, and chia seeds, have anti-inflammatory properties that benefit gut health.

6. Healthy Fats: Incorporating healthy fats from sources like avocados, nuts, and olive oil can support nutrient absorption and gut function.

7. Bone Broth: Bone broth is rich in nutrients that support gut lining health, including collagen, amino acids, and minerals.

8. Herbal Teas: Some herbal teas, like peppermint and ginger tea, have soothing properties that can help ease digestive discomfort.

4.1.2 Foods to Avoid for Gut Health

1. Processed Foods: Highly processed foods often contain artificial additives, preservatives, and unhealthy fats that can disrupt gut health and contribute to inflammation.

2. Added Sugars: Excessive sugar intake can negatively impact the gut microbiome, promoting the growth of harmful bacteria and yeast.

3. Artificial Sweeteners: Some artificial sweeteners may disrupt gut bacteria and cause digestive discomfort in some individuals.

4. High-Fat and Fried Foods: While healthy fats are beneficial, excessive consumption of high-fat and fried foods can lead to digestive issues and inflammation.

5. Red Meat: Consuming large amounts of red meat has been associated with an increased risk of certain gut disorders.

6. Gluten (for Some Individuals): Gluten, found in wheat, barley, and rye, can be problematic for individuals with gluten sensitivity or celiac disease.

7. Excessive Alcohol: Heavy alcohol consumption can disrupt the gut microbiome and damage the gut lining.

8. Artificial Additives: Artificial colors, flavors, and preservatives

found in processed foods may have negative effects on gut health.

It's important to note that individual tolerances to certain foods may vary, and some people may be more sensitive to specific dietary components than others. A personalized approach to nutrition, focusing on whole, unprocessed foods and paying attention to individual reactions, can help promote a healthy gut and overall well-being. If you have specific gut health concerns or dietary restrictions, consulting with a registered dietitian or healthcare professional can be beneficial in tailoring a gut-friendly diet plan.

4.2 Lifestyle and Stress Management

Lifestyle factors, including stress management, have a profound impact on gut health. Chronic stress and certain lifestyle choices can disrupt the balance of the gut microbiome and negatively affect gut function. Adopting healthy lifestyle practices and employing stress reduction techniques can significantly contribute to maintaining a healthy gut. Here's an exploration of the impact of stress on gut health and some effective techniques for stress reduction:

4.2.1 Impact of Stress on Gut Health

The gut and the brain are closely connected through the gut-brain axis, a complex bidirectional communication system. Stress, whether acute or chronic, can influence gut function and the gut microbiome in several ways:

1. Gut Permeability: Chronic stress can lead to increased gut permeability, often referred to as "leaky gut." This means that the lining of the intestine becomes more permeable, allowing substances that should not enter the bloodstream, such as undigested food particles and toxins, to pass through. This can trigger inflammation and disrupt gut health.

2. Gut Motility: Stress can affect gut motility, leading to changes in bowel movements. Some individuals may experience diarrhea or constipation during periods of heightened stress.

3. Gut Microbiome: Stress can alter the composition of the gut microbiome, leading to an imbalance of beneficial and harmful bacteria. This imbalance can affect gut health and overall well-being.

4. Immune Function: Chronic stress can suppress the immune system, making individuals more susceptible to gut infections and other digestive issues.

4.2.2 Techniques for Stress Reduction

Reducing stress is essential for supporting gut health and overall wellness. Implementing stress reduction techniques can positively influence the gut-brain axis and promote a healthier gut. Here are some effective strategies for managing stress:

1. Mindfulness Meditation: Mindfulness practices involve focusing on the present moment without judgment. Regular meditation can reduce stress and anxiety levels, benefiting gut health.

2. Deep Breathing Exercises: Deep breathing exercises, such as diaphragmatic breathing, can activate the body's relaxation response and help reduce stress.

3. Physical Activity: Regular physical activity, such as walking, yoga, or dancing, can be an effective way to manage stress and support gut health.

4. Adequate Sleep: Prioritize getting enough sleep, as sleep deprivation

can contribute to increased stress and negatively impact gut health.

5. Social Support: Maintaining social connections and seeking support from friends, family, or support groups can help alleviate stress.

6. Limiting Caffeine and Alcohol: Excessive caffeine and alcohol consumption can contribute to stress and disrupt gut health. Moderation is key.

7. Hobbies and Creativity: Engaging in hobbies and creative activities can provide a positive outlet for stress and promote relaxation.

8. Setting Boundaries: Learn to say no and set healthy boundaries to reduce feelings of overwhelm and stress.

9. Time Management: Effective time management can help reduce stress by creating a sense of control over daily tasks and commitments.

10. Seeking Professional Help: If stress becomes overwhelming and affects daily life, consider seeking support from a therapist or counselor.

By incorporating stress reduction techniques into daily life, individuals can positively impact their gut health and overall well-being. Adopting a holistic approach that addresses both dietary and lifestyle factors can lead to improved gut health and support a healthier, more balanced gut microbiome.

CHAPTER 5

Gut Health and Women's Health

5.1 Hormones and Gut Health

Hormones play a crucial role in regulating various bodily functions, including gut health. The intricate relationship between hormones and the gut is known as the gut-hormone axis. Hormones can influence gut motility, gut permeability, and the composition of the gut microbiome. For women, fluctuations in hormones during different life stages, such as the menstrual cycle and menopause, can impact gut health in various ways:

Estrogen: Estrogen, one of the primary female sex hormones, has been linked to gut health. During the menstrual cycle, estrogen levels fluctuate, and these changes can affect gut motility, leading to constipation or diarrhea for some women. Additionally, estrogen has been shown to influence gut permeability, potentially affecting gut inflammation and immune responses.

Progesterone: Progesterone is another key female sex hormone that influences the gut. During the menstrual cycle, progesterone levels increase, and this hormone can slow down gut motility, leading to bloating and a feeling of fullness.

Gut Microbiome: Hormonal fluctuations can also impact the gut microbiome composition. Estrogen, in particular, may affect the growth and activity of certain gut bacteria, potentially influencing gut health.

Stress Hormones: Stress hormones, such as cortisol, can also have an impact on gut health. Chronic stress can disrupt the gut-hormone axis and contribute to gut issues, such as irritable bowel syndrome (IBS).

It's important to recognize that the relationship between hormones and gut health can be complex and individualized. Some women may experience significant gut changes during certain points in their menstrual cycle, while others may not notice as much of an impact. Additionally, hormone-related gut issues can vary widely among women.

5.2 Gut Health During Menstruation and Menopause

1. Gut Health During Menstruation:

- Premenstrual Syndrome (PMS): Some women may experience digestive issues, such as bloating, constipation, or diarrhea, during the premenstrual phase due to hormonal fluctuations.

- Food Cravings: Hormonal changes during menstruation can lead to food cravings, especially for sugary and high-fat foods, which can negatively impact gut health if consumed in excess.

- Gut Microbiome: Studies have shown that the gut microbiome may change during the menstrual cycle, particularly in response to hormonal fluctuations.

2. Gut Health During Menopause:

- Hormonal Changes: During menopause, the decline in estrogen levels can impact gut health. Changes in estrogen levels may lead to alterations in gut motility, gut permeability, and the gut microbiome.

- Digestive Issues: Menopausal women may experience digestive symptoms such as bloating, gas, and changes in bowel habits.

- Weight Management: Menopausal women may face challenges with weight management, which can affect gut health and overall well-being.

Maintaining Gut Health During Different Life Stages:

1. Diet and Nutrition: Adopting a gut-friendly diet with plenty of fiber, fermented foods, and prebiotics can

support gut health during different life stages.

2. Stress Management: Managing stress through relaxation techniques, meditation, or regular physical activity can positively impact gut health.

3. Probiotics: Incorporating probiotic-rich foods or supplements can help maintain a balanced gut microbiome.

4. Hydration: Staying hydrated is crucial for gut health and overall digestion.

5. Seeking Professional Advice: If gut issues persist or significantly impact daily life, seeking guidance from a healthcare professional can be beneficial.

As women go through different life stages, understanding the connections between hormones, gut health, and overall well-being can help promote a healthier gut and support optimal health throughout the various phases of life.

CHAPTER 6

Gut-Brain Connection for Women

6.1 Understanding the Gut-Brain Axis

The gut-brain axis is a complex bidirectional communication system that connects the gut and the brain. It involves a continuous exchange of signals and information between the central nervous system (the brain and spinal cord) and the enteric nervous system (ENS), which is sometimes referred to as the "second brain" and encompasses the neurons in the gut.

The gut-brain axis is a two-way communication pathway, meaning that signals can travel from the gut to the brain and vice versa. This communication occurs through various pathways, including the nervous system, hormonal signaling, and immune system modulation. The gut and the brain communicate through the vagus nerve, a major nerve that runs between the brain and the abdomen, as well as through the release of neurotransmitters, hormones, and immune factors.

The gut microbiome, the vast community of microorganisms residing in the gastrointestinal tract, also plays a vital role in the gut-brain axis. The gut microbiome produces and interacts with various neuroactive compounds, such as neurotransmitters and short-chain fatty acids, which can influence brain function and behavior.

The gut-brain axis has a profound impact on various physiological processes, including digestion, metabolism, immune function, and emotional regulation. It affects mood, stress responses, and cognitive function. Research has increasingly shown that imbalances in the gut microbiome and disruptions in gut health can contribute to mental health issues, such as anxiety and depression.

6.2 Mental Health and Gut Health

The connection between mental health and gut health is a growing area of research. The gut-brain axis plays a significant role in influencing emotional well-being and mental health. Here are some key aspects of the gut-brain connection as it relates to mental health:

1. Gut Microbiome and Mood: The gut microbiome produces various neurotransmitters, including serotonin and gamma-aminobutyric acid (GABA), which are involved in regulating mood and emotions. Changes in the gut microbiome can impact the production and availability of these neurotransmitters, potentially influencing mood and mental health.

2. Inflammation and Mental Health: An imbalanced gut microbiome can lead to increased gut permeability, allowing harmful substances to enter the

bloodstream. This can trigger systemic inflammation, which has been linked to an increased risk of mood disorders, such as depression.

3. Stress Response: The gut-brain axis is closely linked to the body's stress response. Chronic stress can disrupt the gut microbiome and increase gut permeability, contributing to a negative impact on mental health.

4. Gut Hormones: Hormones produced in the gut, such as ghrelin and leptin, can influence appetite, food intake, and mood.

5. Anxiety and Gut Health: There is evidence suggesting that individuals with gastrointestinal disorders, such as irritable bowel syndrome (IBS), may be more

prone to anxiety and other mental health issues.

6. Probiotics and Mental Health: Some studies have shown that probiotics, beneficial bacteria that support gut health, may have a positive impact on mood and may help reduce symptoms of anxiety and depression.

7. Gut Health and Cognitive Function: Gut health can also influence cognitive function and memory. Inflammation and disruptions in the gut-brain axis may be associated with cognitive impairments and neurodegenerative diseases.

The gut-brain axis underscores the importance of maintaining a healthy gut for optimal mental health and emotional well-being. Prioritizing gut health through a balanced diet, stress management, regular physical activity, and probiotic supplementation, if needed, may have positive effects on mental health and cognitive function. However, it's essential to recognize that mental health is multifactorial, and a comprehensive approach that includes professional support, such as therapy and medical intervention, is essential for individuals experiencing mental health challenges.

CHAPTER 7

Tips for Improving Gut Health

Improving gut health is crucial for overall well-being, and several lifestyle strategies can help support a healthy gut. Here are some tips for promoting gut health:

7.1 Incorporating Probiotics and Prebiotics

- Probiotics: Include probiotic-rich foods in your diet, such as yogurt, kefir, sauerkraut, kimchi, tempeh, and miso. Probiotics are beneficial live bacteria that help maintain a balanced gut microbiome.

- Probiotic Supplements: Consider taking high-quality probiotic supplements if you have specific gut health concerns or if you want to ensure sufficient probiotic intake.

- Prebiotics: Consume prebiotic-rich foods to nourish the beneficial bacteria in your gut. Foods like onions, garlic, bananas, asparagus, and chicory root are excellent sources of prebiotics.

7.2 Importance of Hydration

- Drink plenty of water throughout the day to stay hydrated. Proper hydration supports digestive function and helps prevent constipation.

- Limit excessive consumption of caffeinated and alcoholic beverages, as they can lead to dehydration and potentially disrupt gut health.

7.3 Regular Exercise and Gut Health

- Engage in regular physical activity. Exercise helps maintain gut motility and supports overall digestive health.

- Aim for a combination of cardiovascular exercises and strength training to promote a healthy gut and overall well-being.

- Find activities you enjoy to make exercise a sustainable part of your routine.

Additional Tips for Gut Health:

- Eat a Diverse Diet: Consume a wide variety of plant-based foods, including fruits, vegetables, whole grains, legumes, nuts, and seeds. A diverse diet nourishes the gut microbiome and promotes overall gut health.

- Reduce Processed Foods: Minimize the intake of processed and sugary foods, as they can negatively impact the gut microbiome and lead to inflammation.

- Manage Stress: Practice stress reduction techniques, such as meditation, deep breathing, yoga, or spending time in nature. Chronic stress can disrupt the gut-brain axis and affect gut health.

- Limit Antibiotic Use: Use antibiotics only when necessary and as prescribed by a healthcare professional. Overuse of antibiotics can disrupt the gut microbiome.

- Get Adequate Sleep: Prioritize good sleep hygiene to support gut health and overall well-being. Aim for 7-9 hours of quality sleep per night.

- Avoid Smoking: If you smoke, consider quitting. Smoking can harm the gut lining and negatively impact gut health.

- Chew Food Thoroughly: Practice mindful eating and chew food thoroughly to aid digestion and nutrient absorption.

- Seek Professional Advice: If you have persistent gut issues or specific concerns about gut health, consult with a registered dietitian or healthcare professional for personalized guidance and support.

By implementing these tips and adopting a holistic approach to gut health, you can promote a balanced gut microbiome, improve digestion, and support overall health and vitality. Remember that individual responses to lifestyle changes may vary, so be patient and consistent in your efforts to achieve better gut health.

CHAPTER 8

Digestive Disorders and Women

8.1 Irritable Bowel Syndrome (IBS)

Irritable Bowel Syndrome (IBS) is a common functional digestive disorder that affects the large intestine (colon). It is characterized by a group of symptoms, including abdominal pain, bloating, and changes in bowel habits (diarrhea, constipation, or alternating between both). IBS is more prevalent in women, and it often begins in early adulthood. The exact cause of IBS is not fully understood, but it is believed to be a combination of factors, including gut hypersensitivity, abnormal gut motility, and disturbances in the gut-brain axis.

Key points about IBS in women:

1. Prevalence: IBS affects about twice as many women as men. The reasons for this gender difference are not entirely clear, but hormonal fluctuations and differences in pain perception may play a role.

2. Hormonal Influence: Hormones, particularly estrogen, have been suggested to influence IBS symptoms in women. Some women experience changes in symptoms during different phases of their menstrual cycle, with worsening symptoms during menstruation.

3. Pregnancy and Menopause:
    Pregnancy and menopause may
    also impact IBS symptoms due to
    hormonal changes during these life
    stages.

4. Stress and Anxiety: Stress and
    anxiety can exacerbate IBS
    symptoms. Women are more likely
    to experience stress and anxiety,
    which can contribute to IBS flare-
    ups.

Treatment for IBS often involves
dietary modifications, stress
management, and lifestyle changes.
Working with a healthcare provider,
such as a gastroenterologist or a
registered dietitian, can help develop
a personalized treatment plan to
manage IBS symptoms effectively.

8.2 Inflammatory Bowel Disease (IBD)

Inflammatory Bowel Disease (IBD) is a chronic condition characterized by inflammation of the gastrointestinal tract. The two main types of IBD are Crohn's disease and ulcerative colitis. While IBD affects both men and women, some differences exist in how the disease presents and affects women:

1. Prevalence: Studies have shown that IBD affects slightly more women than men, though the reasons for this difference are not entirely clear.

2. Pregnancy: Women with IBD may face unique challenges during pregnancy. The disease itself can influence fertility, and women with active IBD may experience

complications during pregnancy.
However, with proper
management and medical care,
most women with IBD can have
successful pregnancies and healthy
babies.

3. Menstrual Cycle: Some women
   with IBD may experience changes
   in disease activity during different
   phases of their menstrual cycle,
   with possible symptom worsening
   during menstruation.

4. Hormonal Therapy: Some women
   with IBD may receive hormonal
   therapies for various medical
   conditions. It's essential for
   women with IBD to work closely
   with their healthcare providers,
   including gastroenterologists and
   gynecologists, to ensure that
   hormonal therapies do not

negatively affect their IBD management.

Management of IBD typically involves a combination of medications, lifestyle modifications, and sometimes surgery. The treatment plan is individualized based on the type and severity of the disease. Regular monitoring by healthcare providers is crucial to manage IBD effectively and prevent complications.

Both IBS and IBD can significantly impact a woman's quality of life, and seeking early medical attention and appropriate care is essential for symptom management and overall well-being. Women with symptoms suggestive of digestive disorders should consult with a healthcare professional for an accurate diagnosis and tailored treatment plan.

CHAPTER 9

Gut Health and Immunity

9.1 The Role of the Gut in Immune Function

The gut plays a crucial role in immune function, and its health is closely linked to the overall strength of the immune system. The gastrointestinal tract is the largest immune organ in the body and is home to a vast community of beneficial bacteria known as the gut microbiome. The interaction between the gut microbiome, gut lining, and the immune system is essential for maintaining a well-balanced and robust immune response.

Key points about the role of the gut in immune function:

1. Gut-Associated Lymphoid Tissue (GALT): The gut contains a significant portion of the body's immune cells, including lymphocytes, which are vital for defending against infections and pathogens.

2. Gut Barrier Function: The gut lining serves as a physical barrier that prevents harmful substances, such as pathogens and toxins, from entering the bloodstream. A healthy gut lining helps maintain gut integrity and supports optimal immune function.

3. Gut Microbiome: The gut microbiome plays a critical role in training and modulating the immune system. Beneficial gut bacteria help educate immune cells and promote immune tolerance, preventing unnecessary inflammation and immune responses to harmless substances.

4. Immune Regulation: The gut microbiome helps regulate the immune system, ensuring that it responds appropriately to infections while avoiding overreacting to harmless antigens, reducing the risk of autoimmune diseases.

5. Immunoglobulin A (IgA): The gut is a primary site for producing IgA, an essential antibody that helps protect the body from

infections by neutralizing pathogens.

6. Immune Memory: The gut is involved in developing immune memory, a crucial process that allows the immune system to recognize and respond more efficiently to previously encountered pathogens.

9.2 Boosting Immunity through Gut Health

Maintaining a healthy gut is essential for supporting a robust immune system. Here are some strategies to promote gut health and boost immunity:

1. Balanced Diet: Consume a nutrient-rich and diverse diet with plenty of fruits, vegetables, whole

grains, lean proteins, and healthy fats. These foods provide essential vitamins, minerals, and antioxidants that support both gut health and immune function.

2. Probiotics: Include probiotic-rich foods or supplements to support a healthy gut microbiome. Probiotics introduce beneficial live bacteria that positively influence immune function.

3. Prebiotics: Consume prebiotic-rich foods to nourish the beneficial gut bacteria. Prebiotics are non-digestible fibers that promote the growth of probiotics.

4. Limit Added Sugars: High sugar intake can negatively impact the gut microbiome and suppress immune function. Minimize the

consumption of sugary beverages and processed foods.

5. Manage Stress: Chronic stress can disrupt the gut-brain axis and immune function. Practice stress-reduction techniques, such as meditation, yoga, or spending time in nature.

6. Regular Exercise: Engage in regular physical activity, as it can promote gut health and support immune function.

7. Get Enough Sleep: Prioritize good sleep hygiene to allow the body and immune system to rest and recover.

8. Avoid Excessive Use of Antibiotics: Unnecessary use of antibiotics can disrupt the gut microbiome and affect immune health. Use antibiotics only when

prescribed by a healthcare professional.

9. Hydration: Stay well-hydrated to support digestion and overall gut health.

By prioritizing gut health, individuals can help optimize their immune function and reduce the risk of infections and immune-related disorders. A healthy gut contributes to a well-balanced and robust immune system, supporting overall health and well-being.

CHAPTER 10

Detoxification and Gut Health

10.1 Supporting Natural Detoxification

Detoxification is the process by which the body eliminates toxins and waste products to maintain optimal health. The liver, kidneys, gastrointestinal tract, skin, and respiratory system are the main organs involved in natural detoxification. While supporting the body's natural detoxification processes is essential, it's important to understand that certain "detox" fads or extreme cleansing methods may not be beneficial for gut health and overall well-being. Instead, focusing on healthy lifestyle practices can effectively support natural detoxification and promote gut health:

1. Hydration: Drinking plenty of water helps flush toxins out of the body through urine and sweat. Staying hydrated supports kidney function, an essential component of natural detoxification.

2. Balanced Diet: Consuming a balanced diet rich in fruits, vegetables, whole grains, and lean proteins provides essential nutrients that support the liver's detoxification pathways.

3. High-Fiber Foods: A diet high in fiber helps regulate bowel movements and promotes the

elimination of waste products from the gut.

4. Gut-Friendly Foods: Incorporate probiotic-rich and prebiotic-rich foods to support a healthy gut microbiome. A well-balanced gut microbiome is essential for gut health and overall well-being.

5. Limit Processed Foods: Minimize the intake of processed and unhealthy foods that may burden the liver and contribute to inflammation.

6. Regular Exercise: Physical activity supports circulation, lymphatic flow, and sweating, all of which contribute to natural detoxification.

7. Stress Management: Chronic stress can impact detoxification processes. Engaging in stress-

reduction techniques, such as mindfulness practices or yoga, can support overall well-being.

10.2 Cleanses and Gut Health

Cleanses and extreme detox diets that involve restrictive eating patterns, fasting, or the use of specific supplements have become popular in recent years. However, it's important to approach these practices with caution, as they may not be beneficial for gut health and can even be harmful:

1. Nutrient Deficiencies: Extreme detox diets often lack essential nutrients, which can lead to nutrient deficiencies and negatively impact overall health.

2. Disruption of Gut Microbiome:
    Drastic changes in diet, especially
    those involving excessive use of
    laxatives or fasting, can disrupt the
    gut microbiome and lead to
    imbalances.

3. Dehydration: Some cleanses or
    detox diets may cause dehydration,
    which is detrimental to gut health
    and can lead to other health issues.

4. Weight Fluctuations: Cleanses that
    promote rapid weight loss are
    often not sustainable and may lead
    to weight fluctuations, which can
    affect gut health and metabolism.

5. Potential for Harm: Extreme detox
    methods can put a strain on the
    liver and other organs involved in
    natural detoxification, potentially
    causing harm.

It's crucial to remember that the body is designed to detoxify itself naturally through the organs mentioned earlier. Instead of extreme cleanses, focus on adopting a balanced and sustainable lifestyle that supports the body's natural detoxification processes. If you have concerns about your gut health or are considering a specific detox program, it's advisable to consult with a registered dietitian or healthcare professional to ensure that your approach is safe and appropriate for your individual health needs.

CHAPTER 11

Gut Health Maintenance for Women

11.1 Creating a Gut-Friendly Meal Plan

Maintaining gut health is essential for overall well-being, and women can take specific steps to support a healthy gut through their diet. Here's a guide to creating a gut-friendly meal plan:

1. Include Fiber-Rich Foods: Incorporate a variety of fruits, vegetables, whole grains, legumes,

nuts, and seeds into your meals.
These fiber-rich foods promote
regular bowel movements and
nourish the beneficial gut bacteria.

2. Prioritize Prebiotic Foods:
   Consume prebiotic-rich foods,
   such as onions, garlic, bananas,
   asparagus, and oats, to support the
   growth of beneficial gut bacteria.

3. Add Probiotic Foods: Include
   probiotic-rich foods like yogurt,
   kefir, sauerkraut, kimchi, and miso
   to introduce beneficial live
   bacteria to the gut.

4. Choose Lean Proteins: Opt for lean
   sources of protein such as fish,
   poultry, tofu, and legumes. Protein
   is essential for tissue repair and
   supports a healthy gut lining.

5. Healthy Fats: Include sources of
   healthy fats like avocados, nuts,

seeds, and olive oil. Healthy fats are beneficial for gut health and overall well-being.

6. Limit Added Sugars: Minimize the consumption of foods and beverages with added sugars, as excessive sugar intake can negatively impact the gut microbiome.

7. Moderate Alcohol and Caffeine: Limit alcohol consumption, as excessive alcohol can disrupt the gut microbiome. Moderation is also key when it comes to caffeine intake.

8. Hydration: Stay well-hydrated by drinking plenty of water throughout the day. Proper hydration supports digestion and gut health.

9. Mindful Eating: Practice mindful eating, chewing food thoroughly, and enjoying meals in a relaxed setting. This aids digestion and nutrient absorption.

10. Manage Stress: Incorporate stress-reduction techniques, such as meditation, deep breathing, or yoga, to support gut health and overall well-being.

Sample Gut-Friendly Meal Plan:

Breakfast:

- Overnight oats with chia seeds, topped with fresh berries and a dollop of Greek yogurt (probiotic).

- Herbal tea or green tea.

Lunch:

- Quinoa salad with mixed vegetables, chickpeas (prebiotic), and a lemon-tahini dressing (healthy fats).

- Fermented vegetables like kimchi or sauerkraut (probiotic) on the side.

Snack:

- Carrot sticks with hummus (prebiotic) or a handful of almonds (healthy fats).

Dinner:

- Baked salmon (lean protein) with roasted sweet potatoes and steamed broccoli (fiber-rich).

- Mixed leafy greens salad with a sprinkle of flaxseeds (fiber and healthy fats).

Dessert (optional):

- A small serving of dark chocolate (70% cocoa or higher) for a touch of antioxidants.

Individual dietary needs and preferences vary, so it's important to customize the meal plan to suit your specific requirements. Consulting with a registered dietitian can provide personalized guidance and ensure that your meal plan supports your gut health and overall nutritional needs.

11.2 Long-Term Strategies for Gut Health

Long-term strategies for gut health are essential to maintain a healthy gut and overall well-being. These strategies involve adopting healthy habits and lifestyle choices that support the gut microbiome and digestive function. Here are some long-term strategies for gut health:

1. Balanced and Diverse Diet: Follow a balanced diet rich in a variety of fruits, vegetables, whole grains, lean proteins, and healthy fats. A diverse diet provides a wide range of nutrients and promotes a diverse gut microbiome.

2. Mindful Eating: Practice mindful eating by chewing food thoroughly, eating in a relaxed environment, and paying attention to hunger and fullness cues. Mindful eating supports optimal digestion and nutrient absorption.

3. Regular Probiotics and Prebiotics: Incorporate probiotic-rich foods or supplements to introduce beneficial live bacteria to the gut.

Consume prebiotic-rich foods to nourish the gut microbiome and support the growth of beneficial bacteria.

4. Limit Processed Foods: Minimize the intake of processed and unhealthy foods that may negatively impact the gut microbiome and contribute to inflammation.

5. Manage Stress: Chronic stress can disrupt the gut-brain axis and gut health. Engage in stress-reduction techniques like meditation, yoga, or spending time in nature.

6. Regular Physical Activity: Stay physically active to support gut health and overall well-being. Regular exercise promotes gut motility and a healthy gut microbiome.

7. Sufficient Hydration: Drink plenty of water throughout the day to support digestion and prevent constipation.

8. Avoid Unnecessary Antibiotics: Use antibiotics only when prescribed by a healthcare professional. Unnecessary use of antibiotics can disrupt the gut microbiome.

9. Get Adequate Sleep: Prioritize good sleep hygiene and aim for 7-9 hours of quality sleep each night to support gut health and overall health.

10. Limit Alcohol and Caffeine: Consume alcohol and caffeine in moderation, as excessive intake can negatively impact the gut microbiome.

11. Regular Health Check-ups: Schedule regular health check-ups and screenings to monitor gut health and overall well-being.

12. Listen to Your Body: Pay attention to how your body responds to different foods and lifestyle choices. Everyone's gut health is unique, so it's essential to listen to your body's cues and make adjustments accordingly.

Maintaining gut health is a lifelong journey, and small, consistent changes over time can have a significant impact on gut health and overall wellness. Building healthy habits and taking a holistic approach to gut health will contribute to a balanced gut microbiome and support your overall health and quality of life in the long run. If you have specific gut health concerns or medical conditions,

consult with a healthcare professional
or registered dietitian for personalized
guidance and support.

CHAPTER 12

Embracing a Gut-Healthy Lifestyle

Embracing a gut-healthy lifestyle involves making long-term, sustainable changes that prioritize the well-being of your gastrointestinal tract and overall health. By adopting a holistic approach to gut health, you can support the balance of your gut microbiome and promote optimal digestion and immune function. Here are some key components of a gut-healthy lifestyle:

1. Balanced Diet: Follow a balanced and varied diet that includes a wide range of nutrient-rich foods. Emphasize fruits, vegetables,

whole grains, lean proteins, and healthy fats. This diverse diet nourishes the gut microbiome and provides essential nutrients for overall health.

2. Mindful Eating: Practice mindful eating by eating slowly, savoring your meals, and paying attention to hunger and fullness cues. Avoid distractions while eating to enhance digestion.

3. Probiotics and Prebiotics: Regularly incorporate probiotic-rich foods (e.g., yogurt, kefir, fermented vegetables) and prebiotic-rich foods (e.g., onions, garlic, bananas) to support a balanced gut microbiome.

4. Hydration: Stay well-hydrated by drinking plenty of water throughout the day. Proper

hydration supports digestive function and overall gut health.

5. Manage Stress: Implement stress-reduction techniques such as meditation, deep breathing, yoga, or spending time in nature. Chronic stress negatively affects gut health, so managing stress is crucial.

6. Regular Exercise: Engage in regular physical activity to support gut motility, reduce inflammation, and promote a healthy gut microbiome.

7. Limit Processed Foods: Minimize the consumption of processed and unhealthy foods, as they can negatively impact the gut microbiome and overall health.

8. Adequate Sleep: Prioritize good sleep hygiene and aim for 7-9

hours of quality sleep each night to
support gut health and overall
well-being.

9. Limit Alcohol and Caffeine:
    Consume alcohol and caffeine in
    moderation, as excessive intake
    can disrupt the gut microbiome.

10. Avoid Unnecessary Antibiotics:
    Use antibiotics only when
    prescribed by a healthcare
    professional. Overuse of
    antibiotics can disturb the gut
    microbiome.

11. Regular Health Check-ups:
    Schedule regular health check-ups
    to monitor gut health and overall
    well-being. Discuss any gut-
    related concerns with a healthcare
    professional.

12. Listen to Your Body: Pay attention
    to how your body responds to

different foods and lifestyle choices. Everyone's gut health is unique, so tailor your lifestyle choices based on your individual needs.

13. Seek Professional Advice: If you have specific gut health concerns or medical conditions, consult with a healthcare professional or registered dietitian for personalized guidance and support.

Embracing a gut-healthy lifestyle is a journey, and small changes made consistently over time can have a significant impact on gut health and overall wellness. Prioritize self-care and make choices that support the balance of your gut microbiome, as it is an essential foundation for maintaining optimal health and vitality.